The author

Francisco Javier García Peña

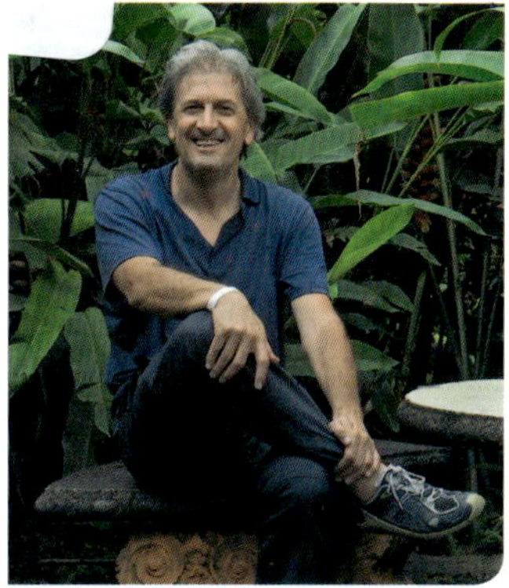

Graduate in Biological Science (1982) and veterinary [illegible] (1986) from the Universidad Complutense de Madrid, Spain. Currently working as a public health inspector (products for human consumption) at the Barajas Airport Border Inspection Post, Madrid. Head of the Bacteriology–2 Department of the Central Veterinary-Animal Health Laboratory (Spanish Ministry of Agriculture and Fisheries, Food and the Environment) in Algete, Madrid for 25 years (1992–2017). Member of GEMAS (Grupo de Estudio de la Medicina y Conservación de Animales Silvestres), a study group for indigenous wild animal medicine and conservation.

TABLE OF CONTENTS

Major characteristics of the genus *Leptospira*

Leptospires are helically coiled, corkscrew-shaped bacteria, characterised by a high degree of motility, a small diameter (0.1 μm) and 6–20 μm long, with hooked ends. They stain poorly with aniline dyes, despite being Gram–negative. Therefore, a darkfield microscope must be used to observe them.

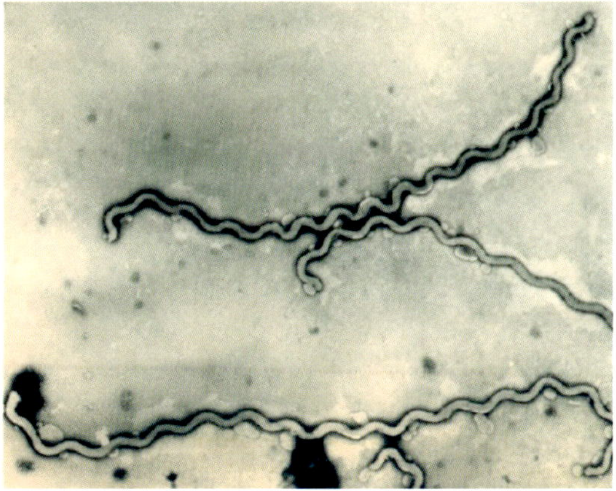

Figure 1. Electron microscopy of *Leptospira* spp.

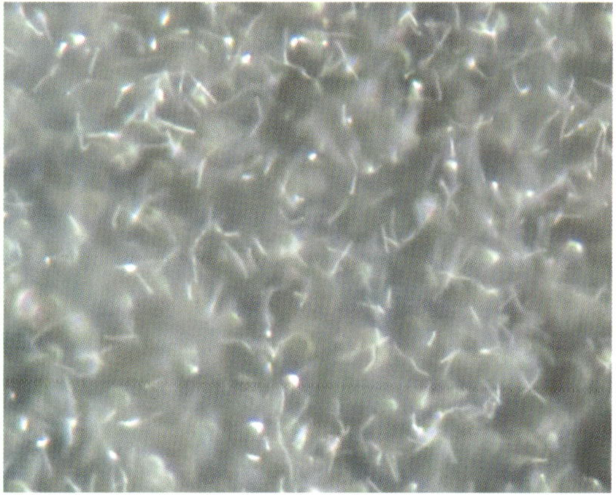

Figure 2. Darkfield microscopy (x150) of *Leptospira* spp. culture.

Table 1. Main characteristics of genus *Leptospira* metabolism, growth and survival outside the host.

Metabolic characteristics	• Obligate aerobic bacteria. • Carbon and energy source: β-oxidation of long-chain fatty acids (longer than 15 carbons). • Nitrogen source: ammonium ions. • Cytochrome c oxidase and catalase activity. • Saprophytic species synthesise purines and pyrimidines, and grow in the presence of 8-azaguanine, but not the pathogenic species.
Growth characteristics	• Optimum temperature for growth: 28–30 °C. • Optimum pH for growth: 7.2–7.6. • Non-pathogenic saprophytic species grow at 11–13 °C. • Division or multiplication time: 6–8 hours for pathogenic species and 4–5 hours for saprophytic species.

Survival outside the host	• Very sensitive to pH, especially acidity. Rapid bacterial death at pH <5.8 and pH >8.0.
	• Very sensitive to desiccation and direct sunlight.
	• Survive longest at temperatures ≤25 °C.
	• Sensitive to chemical disinfectants and detergents.
	• Survival in boar semen: no data available. Survival in bull semen at 2 °C:
	  – 58 days without antibiotics.
	  – 29 days with antibiotics.
	• Survival in urine:
	  – Undiluted: a few hours.
	  – Mixed with liquid faeces: up to 2 months.

Taxonomy

The genus *Leptospira* originally consisted of two species: *Leptospira biflexa*, comprising all free-living strains, and *Leptospira interrogans*, containing all pathogenic strains. Twenty-two species have been described to date, including pathogenic and free-living species, and certain species that include opportunistic pathogenic strains.

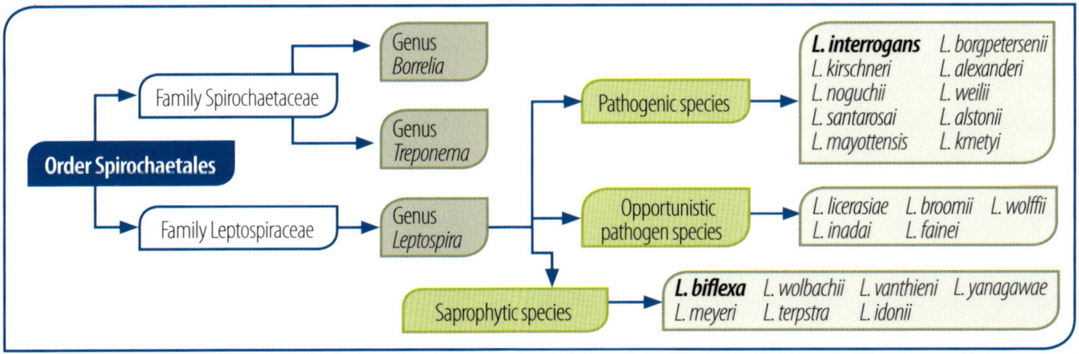

Figure 3. Taxonomic classification of the genus *Leptospira*.

The basic taxonomic unit used to classify *Leptospira* is the serovar, and more than 250 of these have been described. Classification into serovars is based on antigenic criteria (outer membrane lipopolysaccharides).

Finally, serovars sharing common antigens are grouped into artificial taxons, called serogroups. Using this method, the 250+ serovars are grouped in 24 serogroups.

Leptospira taxonomy is complex, because there is no correlation between species and serogroup, so:

- Serovars in the same serogroup can belong to different species. For example, *L. interrogans* serovar Pomona and *L. kirschneri* serovar Mozdok belong to the same serogroup Pomona.
- Serovars in different serogroups can belong to the same species. For example, serovar Pomona in the serogroup Pomona and serovar Icterohaemorrhagiae in the serogroup Icterohaemorrhagiae both belong to the species *L. interrogans*.

Table 2. Definition of the various taxa within the genus *Leptospira* and examples of the classification of serovar Bratislava in each.

Taxon	Definition	Example
Genomospecies	Two *Leptospira* strains belong to the same species when DNA–DNA hybridisation tests demonstrate a level of hybridisation of at least: • 70 % at optimum temperature (55 °C) with at least 5 % divergence between the related sequences. • 60 % at a temperature of 70 °C.	*Leptospira interrogans*
Serogroup	A group of serovars that are different but antigenically related and which therefore cross-react serologically to a certain extent.	Australis serogroup
Serovar	Two *Leptospira* strains (A and B) belong to different serovars if, after cross absorption of the hyperimmune sera with adequate amounts of the heterologous antigen (antiserum A + strain B and antiserum B + strain A), 10 % or more of the homologous titre remains in at least 1 of the 2 antisera in repeated tests.	Serovar Bratislava
Strain / genotype	Isolates that are antigenically similar, but genetically different.	Genotype B1 Genotype B2a Genotype B2b

For practical purposes, the terms serovar and serogroup are always used, because they are relevant to epidemiology, clinical signs, diagnosis and control of infection. Species names are of secondary importance, and only relevant on a taxonomic level.

Pigs as hosts for *Leptospira* spp.

Pigs can act as maintenance hosts for one or more serovars of *Leptospira* species. These serovars are said to be adapted to the pig as a host species. Pigs are termed accidental hosts for serovars which are non-adapted to the pig as a host. These concepts and their implications for various aspects of infection are shown in Fig. 1 and Table 1 respectively.

Maintenance and accidental hosts can vary between ecosystems and geographical regions. An animal species may be a reservoir for several serovars and different animal species may host the same serovar. Some of the most representative serovars and their maintenance hosts are shown in Table 2.

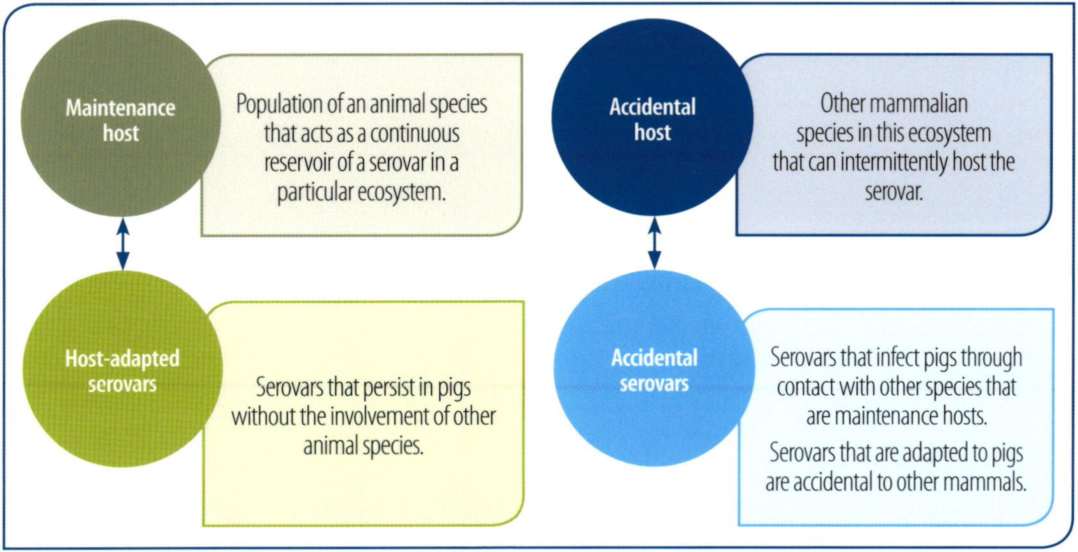

Figure 1. Concept of maintenance host, accidental host, host-adapted serovar and accidental serovar.

Table 1. Characteristics of infection by host-adapted and accidental serovars. Although serovar Pomona is typically adapted to pigs as hosts, it actually displays characteristics of both types of infection.

Features of the infection	Host-adapted serovar		Accidental serovar
	Bratislava	Pomona	
Transmission	Intraspecific		Interspecific
Susceptibility	High		Low
Pathogenicity	Low	Average	High
Clinical forms	Chronic (reproductive disorders)		Acute in young animals (haemolytic crisis), and abortion
Leptospiruria	Mild	Severe and very prolonged	Days to weeks
Persistence in the genitals	Yes	No	
Presentation	Endemic		Sporadic
% Population seropositive	High and increases with age		Low
Immune response	Low antibody titres	High antibody titres	
Diagnosis	Herd level: difficult	Individual level: practical and easy	
Control by vaccination	Relatively ineffective at preventing infection	Very effective at preventing infection	

Table 2. Maintenance hosts and prevalence of host-adapted and accidental serovars in pigs in Spain.

Serovar	Maintenance host	% Positive farms (290 tested)	% Positive serum (5088 tested)
Host-adapted			
Bratislava	Pigs, hedgehogs, horses, dogs and rodents	86.2 %	34.3 %
Pomona	Pigs, wild boar, rodents and skunks	3.1 %	1.1 %
Tarassovi	Pigs and wild animals	2.8 %	0.2 %
Accidental			
Icterohaemorrhagiae	Rodents	15.5 %	2.4 %
Canicola	Dogs	12.8 %	1.3 %
Grippotyphosa	Rodents	3.4 %	0.3 %
Hardjo	Cattle and sheep	0.3 %	0.02 %

Pigs as maintenance hosts

Pigs are considered maintenance hosts for strains of the serovars Pomona, Tarassovi and Bratislava. Farms are usually infected by host-adapted serovars through the introduction of infected sows or boars. Serovar Bratislava also enters via contaminated semen.

In outdoor pig farming, direct contact with wild boar (maintenance hosts for serovar Pomona and probably also Bratislava) or their urine, or other wild animals, such as hedgehogs or skunks (maintenance hosts for the serovars Bratislava and Pomona respectively) is also important.

Pigs as accidental hosts

Pigs can also be infected by serovars maintained by other species, both domestic and wild, and thereby become accidental hosts for the infection. Serovars Icterohaemorrhagiae, Canicola, Grippotyphosa and Hardjo are cited in the literature as the most common accidental serovars to infect pigs. In these cases, infection is through contact between pigs and the urine of maintenance hosts for these serovars.

Wild animals, mainly different species of rodent, are the most important reservoirs for the various accidental serovars in pigs. Infection with these serovars is more common in outdoor pigs, as contact with the contaminated urine of these animals is more likely.

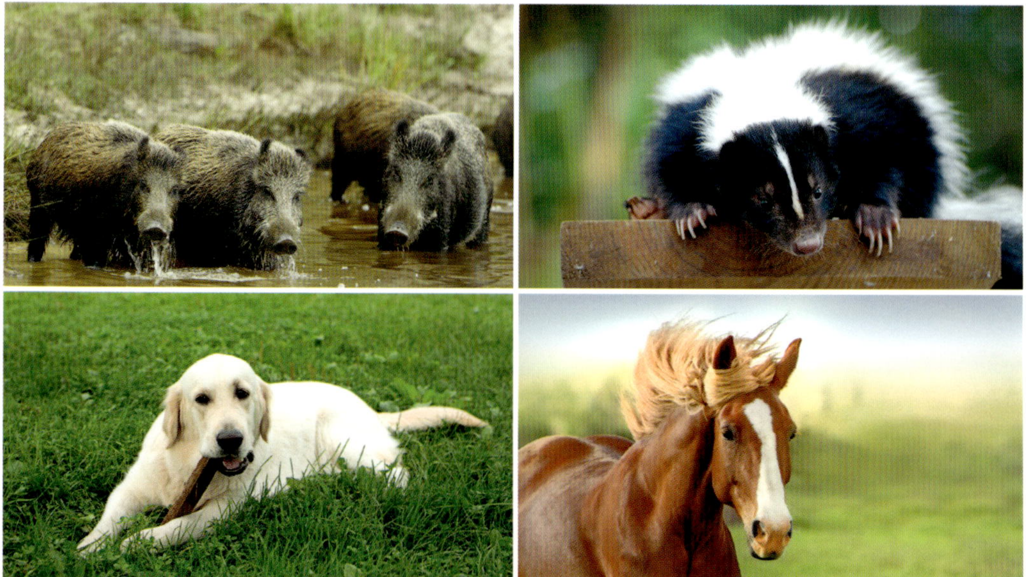

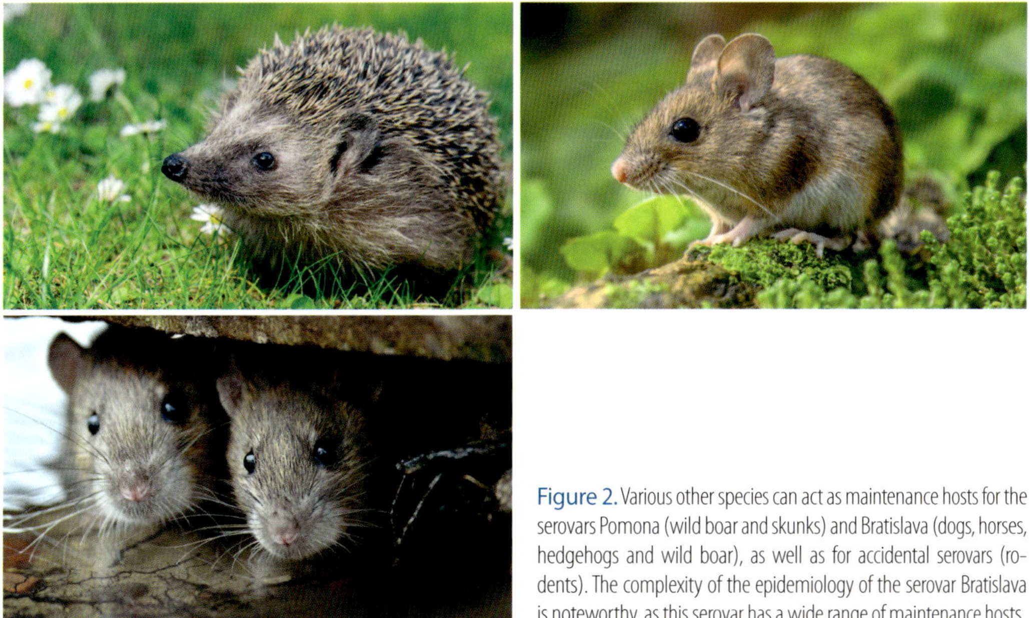

Figure 2. Various other species can act as maintenance hosts for the serovars Pomona (wild boar and skunks) and Bratislava (dogs, horses, hedgehogs and wild boar), as well as for accidental serovars (rodents). The complexity of the epidemiology of the serovar Bratislava is noteworthy, as this serovar has a wide range of maintenance hosts.

Geographical distribution and prevalence

Geographical distribution

Leptospirosis is a cosmopolitan disease, so any pathogenic serovar should theoretically be able to infect pigs. However, the concept of "nidality" has been used to describe the localised nature of this disease, based on the fact that in any particular country or geographical region only a small number of these serovars are endemic. The serovar Tarassovi has been described in pigs in Eastern Europe, Vietnam, Cuba and India, but is insignificant in Western Europe, and serovar Pomona is very important in the Americas, Australia and New Zealand, and Central and Eastern Europe, but few cases have been described in Western Europe. The United Kingdom is considered to be free of this serovar. Serovars such as Bratislava and Icterohaemorrhagiae, however, are found worldwide.

Prevalence

Seroprevalence of the disease varies considerably between countries and even between different regions in the same country.

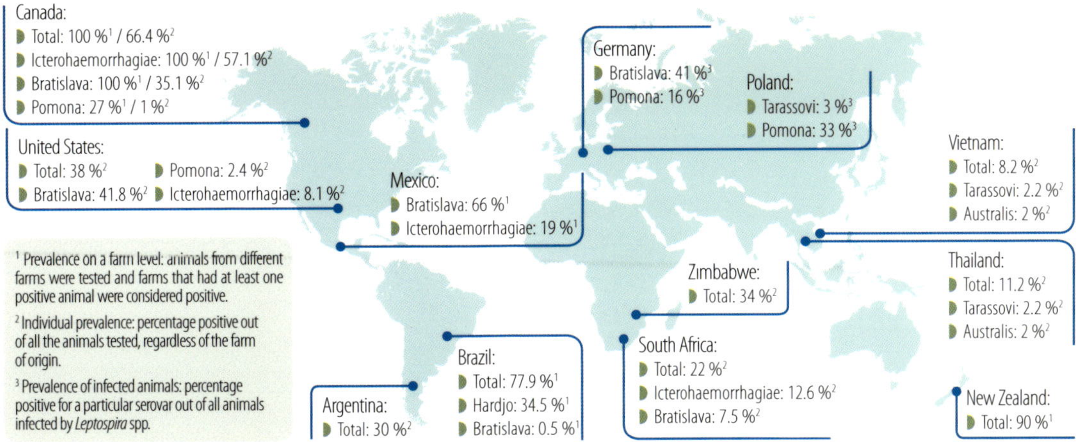

Figure 3. Prevalence of leptospirosis and the most representative serovars in different countries.

Sources of infection, transmission and risk factors

The main sources of infection are urine, placenta, aborted foetuses and vaginal discharge from infected animals, as well as water, grazing land and material contaminated with infected fluids. In the case of serovar Bratislava, semen from infected boars can be an important source of infection.

Direct horizontal transmission is the most common method of transmission for host-adapted serovars. Droplets of urine from animals with leptospiruria can contain large numbers of serovar Pomona and Tarassovi leptospires. These droplets are dispersed some metres from the urinating animal and can infect any animals nearby via the conjunctiva or through inhalation.

Although the serovar Bratislava is also excreted in the urine, the leptospiruria tends to be less severe and of shorter duration. Sexual transmission during mating or artificial insemination is thought to be the main route of transmission. Although no studies have been carried out into excretion or survival times in pig semen, strains have been isolated that persist for long periods in the testicles, prostate gland, seminal vesicles and bulbourethral glands.

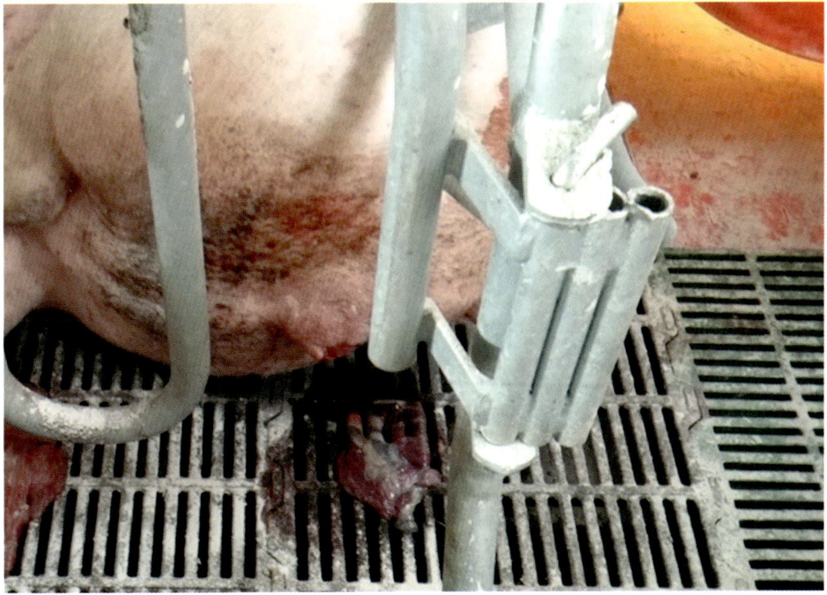

Figure 4. Placental remains from aborted sows are an important source of infection.

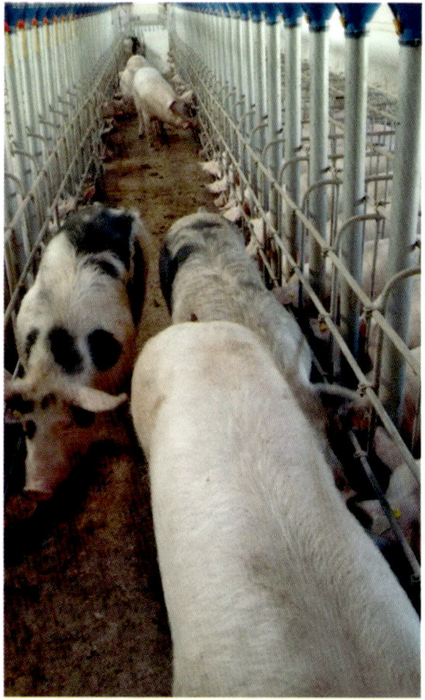

Figure 5. Introduction of infected breeding boars is one of the most common ways that infection is brought into the farm.

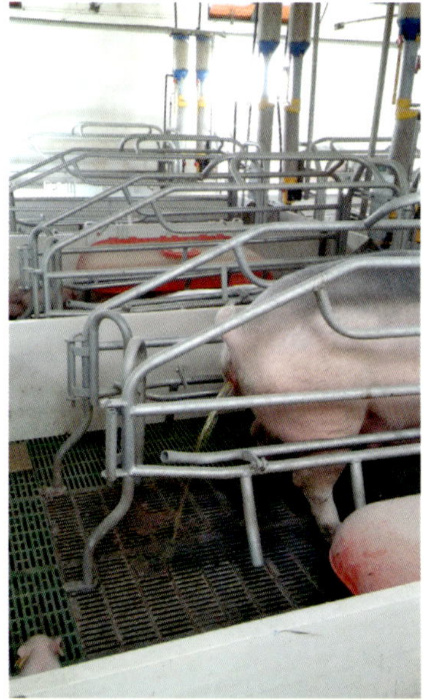

Figure 6. The main transmission route for serovars Pomona and Tarassovi is via droplets of urine from infected animals which splash off the floor and come into contact with the mucosae of uninfected pigs.

Indirect horizontal transmission has a fundamental role in accidental infections, following exposure to an environment contaminated with infective material. Contaminated water and displaceable materials are some of the most important fomites that can facilitate contact between pigs and bacteria.

The possibility of indirect transmission depends to a great extent on survival of the leptospiral organisms in the environment. Factors that prolong survival in the environment are moderate temperatures (25 °C or somewhat lower), a damp environment, neutral or slightly alkaline pH and the presence of organic material, so outbreaks tend to be seasonal, especially in outdoor herds.

Vertical transmission, both across the placenta and in the milk, is also possible. Leptospires can cross the placenta and infect the foetus during the leptospiraemia stage and the foetus can also be infected during birth. Transmission via the milk has only been demonstrated experimentally. Serovar Bratislava has been shown to persist in the retromammary lymph nodes for long periods after abortion.

A small number of studies have been carried out to identify the main risk factors that facilitate horizontal transmission and the following have been observed:

- Use of artificial insemination rather than either natural service or a combination of both.
- No rodent control programme.
- Waterlogged areas.
- Small farms with little technology.
- No quarantine.
- Use of well water rather than mains water.
- High rainfall.

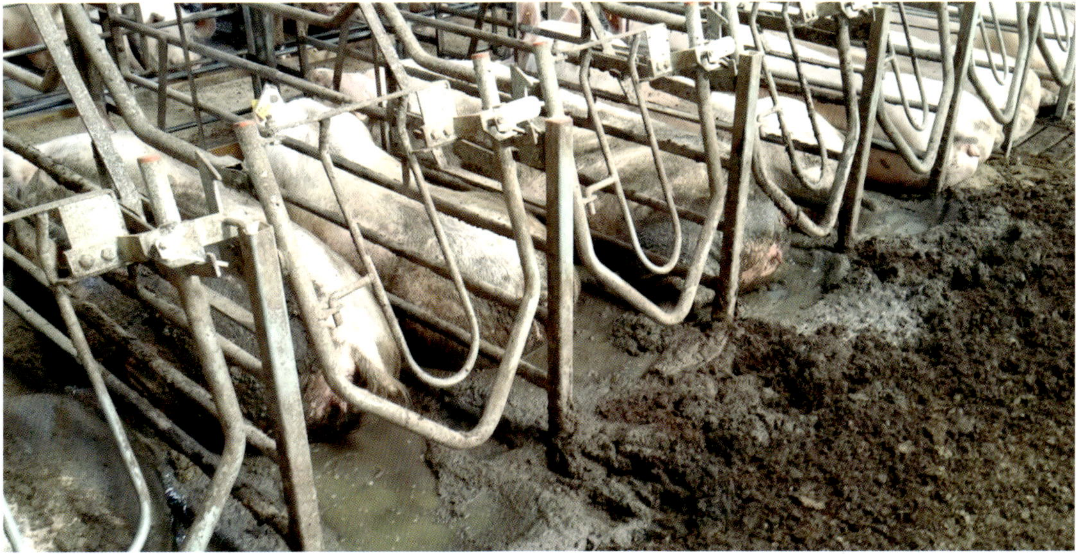

Figure 7. Waterlogged areas and accumulations of organic material prolong leptospire survival in the environment and facilitate transmission.

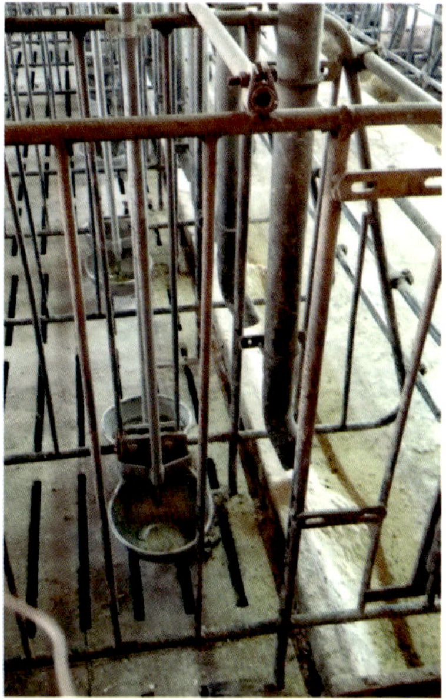

Figure 8. The use of inadequately treated well water is one of the main risk factors enabling leptospirosis to enter the farm.

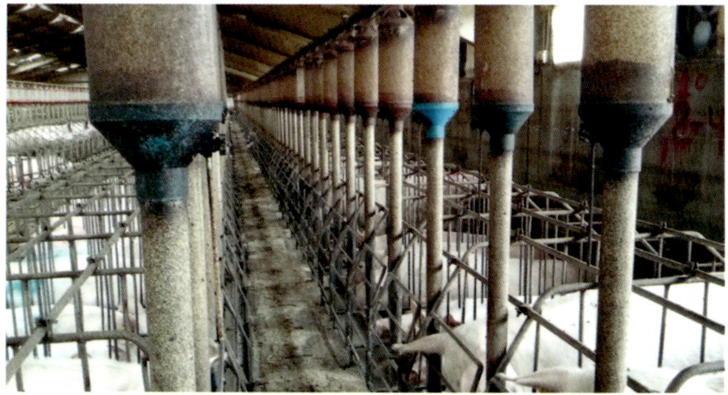

Figure 9. Various studies have found that the risk of infection is lower on large, well-automated farms.

Health implications

Leptospirosis is a zoonosis. However, humans are not maintenance hosts for any serovar, so infection is always accidental. Thus, the prevalence of the disease in humans is merely a reflection of the prevalence in the animal population with which they come into contact. The most common infections in humans are caused by *L. icterohaemorrhagiae*, although those caused by *L. pomona* are also quite common amongst livestock farmers, veterinary surgeons and abattoir workers after handling organs from infected animals or aborted foetuses, or contact with postpartum discharges.

Pathogenesis

Leptospires enter mainly through the conjunctiva and the nasal, oral and genital mucosae, although they can also enter through damaged skin or small cuts and abrasions. Vertical transmission has also been reported.

A leptospiraemic phase occurs 1–2 days after infection and lasts 4–7 days. Agglutinating antibodies can be detected in the serum approximately 5–10 days after infection, and these reach maximum levels about 21 days post infection. This immune response causes leptospires to be eliminated from the blood and most of the organs. However, leptospires can remain in the proximal tubules of the kidneys, and in the reproductive tract in sows and boars.

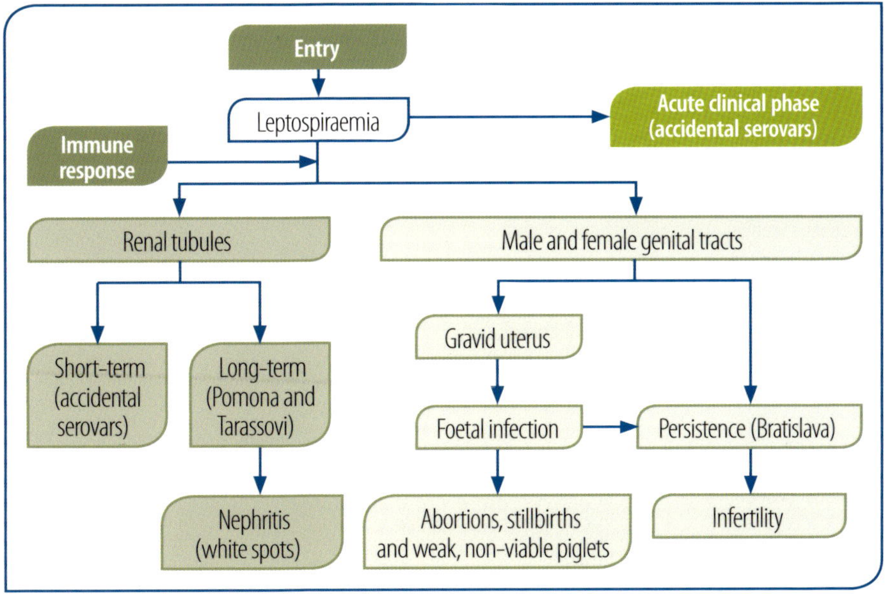

Figure 1. Pathogenesis of leptospirosis according to the serovar involved in the infection.

Clinical presentation

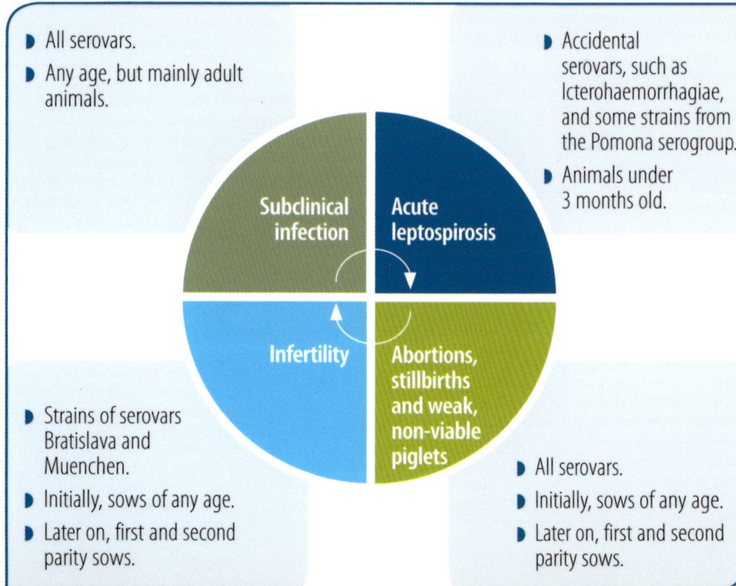

Figure 2. Summary of potential clinical presentations of leptospirosis according to the age of the animal and the serovar involved.

Acute leptospirosis

In animals under 3 months old, infection by accidental serovars and some strains of Pomona can cause severe acute disease with high temperature, jaundice, haemoglobinuria and convulsions. Most animals recover within a week without treatment, but some die.

***Leptospira* infection is usually subclinical in pigs and normally detected by serological testing, but it may present as a serious illness, depending mainly on the serovar involved and the age of the animal infected.**

Chronic leptospirosis

Leptospires colonise and multiply in the kidneys and are excreted in the urine. This stage of leptospiruria is short (2–3 months) in infections caused by accidental serovars, and prolonged with host-adapted serovars, with a leptospiruria sometimes lasting longer than 2 years in the case of Pomona.

In gestating sows, leptospires can cross the placental barrier and infect the foetus during the leptospiraemia stage. Embryonic death, abortion, foetal death and the birth of weak, non-viable piglets usually occur 7–60 days after infection. Sows usually abort shortly after infection with accidental serovars, while abortions and other reproductive disorders can be delayed some weeks or months with host-adapted serovars.

The potential for transplacental infection is lower during the first half of gestation and infection during this period results in embryonic death and reabsorption accompanied by a return to regular or irregular oestrus, or the birth of a small litter with or without mummified foetuses. Foetal infection more usually occurs during the second half of gestation, when the placenta is more permeable, and infection at this stage causes abortions, stillbirths and the birth of weak, non-viable piglets. Infections caused by accidental serovars and the host-adapted serovars Pomona and Tarassovi, do not seem to limit subsequent reproductive performance.

However, serovars Bratislava and Muenchen have been linked to subsequent infertility following an outbreak of abortions. This is because some strains of these serovars can persist in the sow's reproductive tract for up to 5 months after abortion. Persistence in the genital tract has also been reported in boars, so sexual transmission is the main transmission route for these serovars.

The consequences of this persistence in the genitals include regular and irregular returns to oestrus, often accompanied by mucopurulent vaginal discharge 2–3 days before returning, which is reflected in a low conception rate. This infertility tends to last less than 5 months. Although some farmers and veterinary surgeons believe that chronic leptospirosis causes lasting cyclic infertility, there is no evidence to support this theory.

With respect to the evolution of an outbreak, those caused by accidental serovars tend to be sporadic and short-lived due to the very strong immune response they generate and the short renal carrier phase, but infections caused by host-adapted serovars tend to become endemic. Adult sows develop immunity and are protected, although abortions and reproductive problems persist in first and second litter sows that have been raised in isolation since weaning, or are brought onto the farm from a herd which has not been vaccinated or infected.

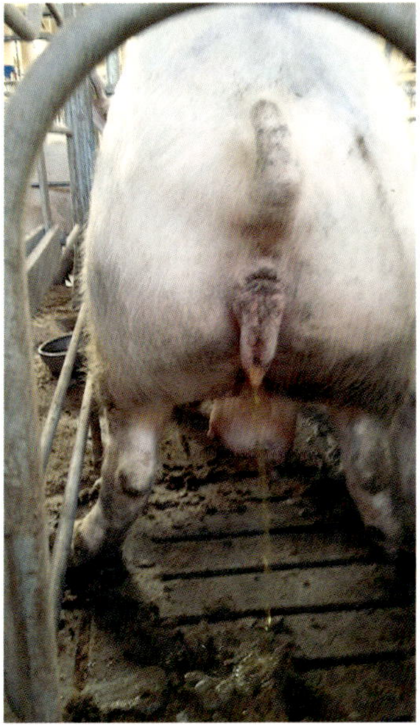

Figure 3. One of the effects of infection is leptospiruria, which can last up to 2 years in the case of serovar Pomona.

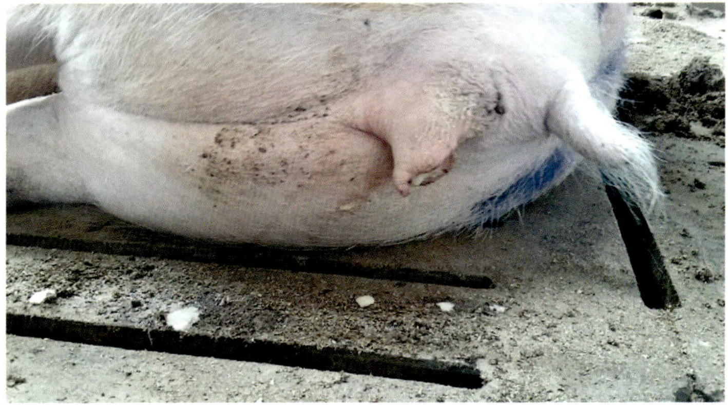

Figure 4. Mucopurulent vaginal discharge is common in infections caused by strains of serovar Bratislava.

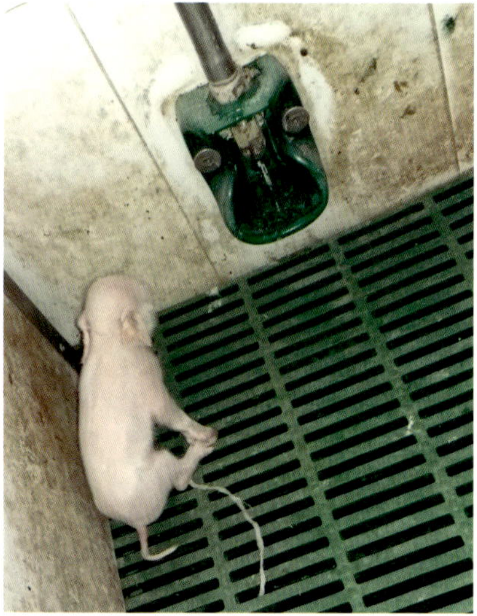

Figure 5. One of the clinical signs of leptospirosis is the birth of weak, non-viable piglets.

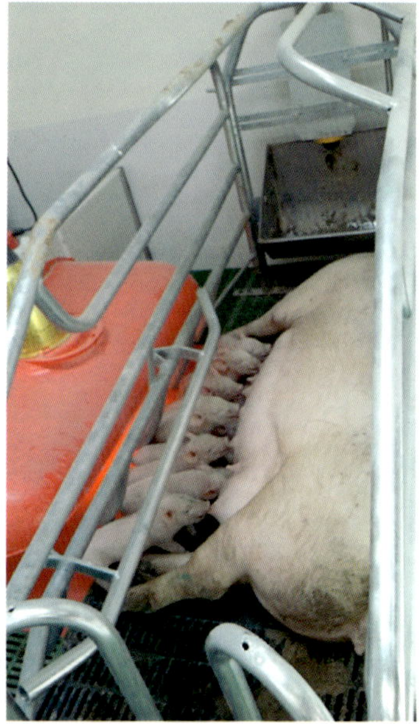

Figure 6. Small litters can be seen in leptospirosis cases, due to its effect on reproduction.

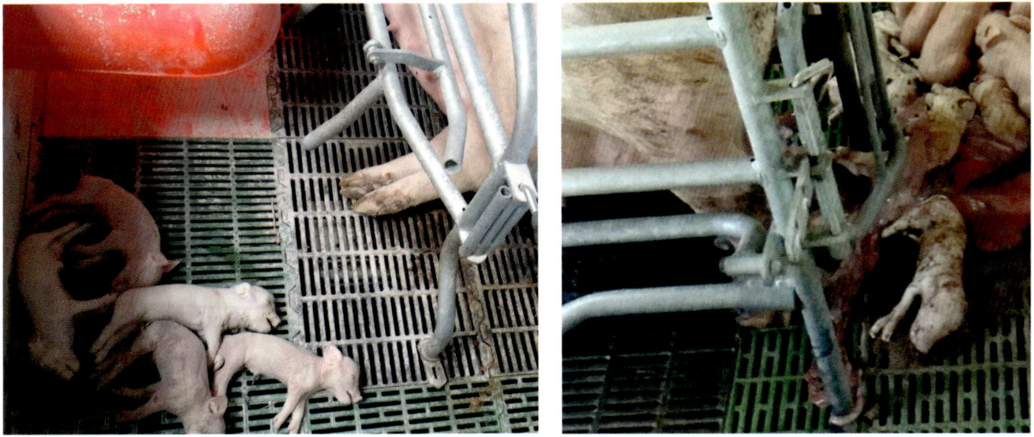

Figure 7. The number of stillborn piglets increases during leptospirosis outbreaks.

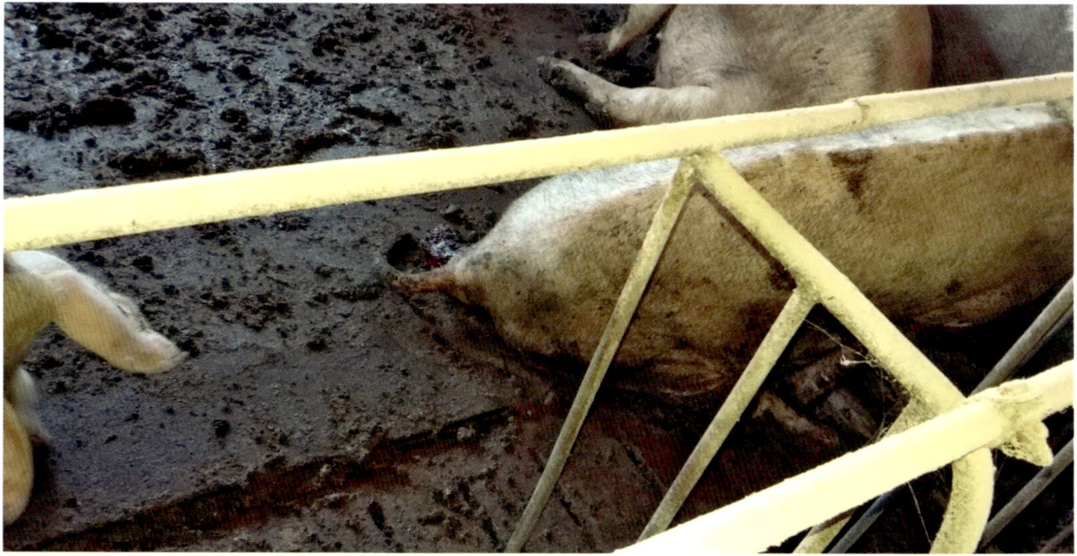

Figure 8. Leptospirosis can cause embryonic losses, especially in serovar Bratislava infections.

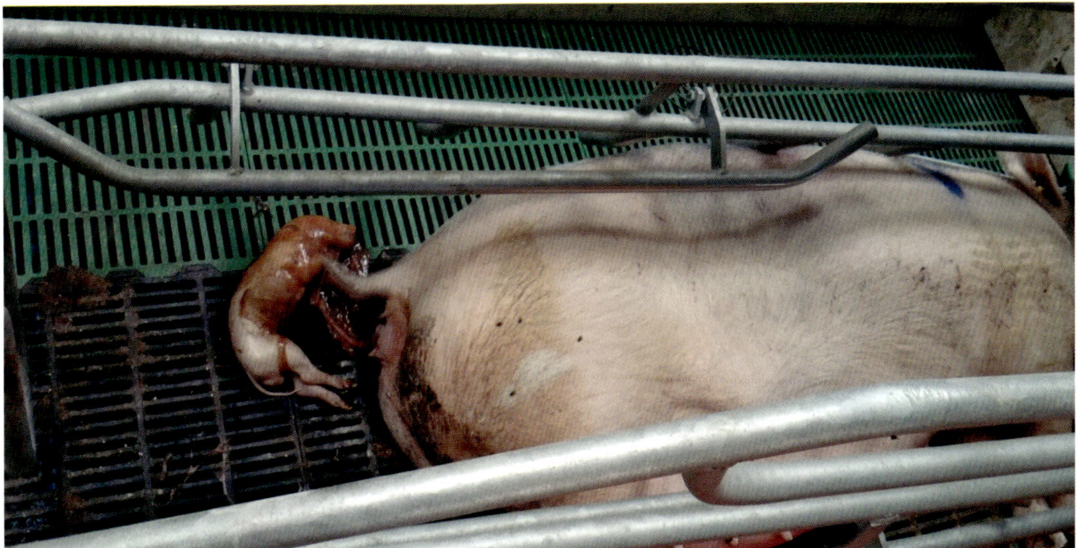

Figure 9. Late abortion is the main clinical sign in a leptospirosis outbreak.

Lesions

In acute cases, dead piglets exhibit jaundice, conjunctival congestion and petechial haemorrhages on the skin and internal organs, mainly the kidneys.

Gross lesions in chronic carrier animals consist of multifocal interstitial nephritis, usually called white-spotted kidneys. This is where irregular whitish areas of up to 1 cm in diameter appear in the renal cortex.

Aborted foetuses can exhibit oedema in various tissues, yellowish or bloody serous fluid in the body cavities and occasional petechial haemorrhages on the skin, renal cortex, liver and lungs. Whitish spots on the liver, caused by focal necrosis, are considered pathognomonic, but are actually only seen in less than 10 % of cases. Aborted foetuses can also be mummified, with pale organs and jaundice.

The placenta usually looks normal, although it can sometimes be thickened and oedematous, or appear necrotic.

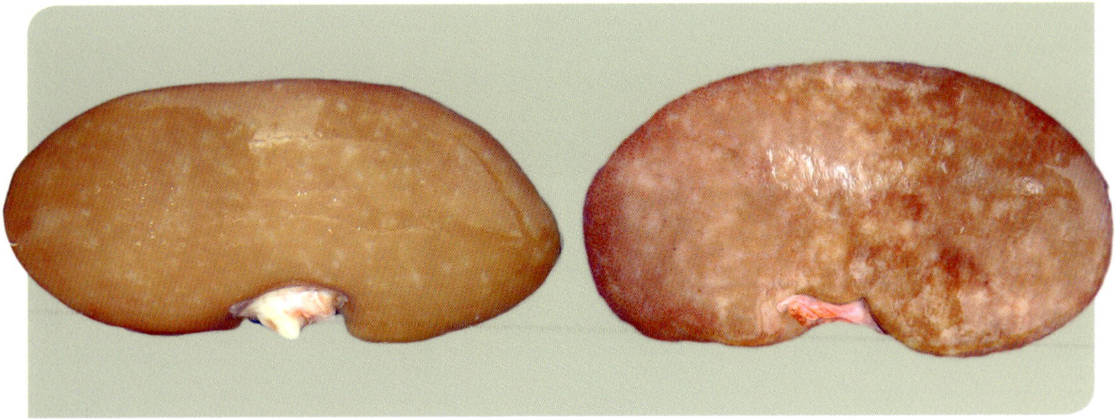

Figure 10. Lesions of interstitial nephritis, possibly due to *Leptospira* infection. Note the whitish areas on the surface of the renal cortex. Images courtesy of Dr Joaquim Segalés, provided by Dr Jorge Martínez (Faculty of Veterinary Medicine, Autonomous University of Barcelona, Spain).

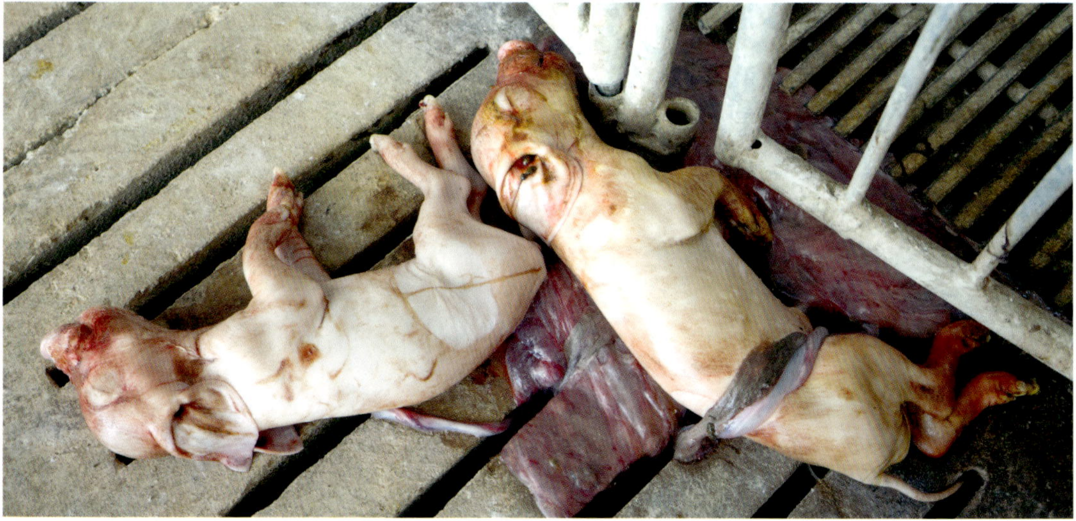

Figure 11. During an outbreak of leptospirosis an increase in the number of mummified foetuses will be observed, with different degrees of mummification according to the stage at which infection has occurred. (Ggamies/shutterstock.com)

Financial impact

It is very difficult to evaluate potential financial losses from an outbreak, as severity can vary considerably. One study carried out in the United States found that the number of piglets weaned/sow/year decreased by about 23 % on farms with chronic, uncontrolled leptospirosis compared with farms that controlled leptospirosis. The production cost per weaned piglet therefore increased by 28.5 % on farms with no control programme.

Another study in the United Kingdom estimated that during an outbreak lasting about 4 months, the number of litters fell by 7 %, and 1.3 fewer piglets were weaned/sow/year. In the case of an endemic disease in first-parity sows, the number of piglets born to the group was calculated to have decreased by 11 %. When feed is medicated in an attempt to improve fertility, feed costs increase by more than €34, and using this feed for a complete reproductive cycle increases the cost per sow by another €17. This cost can be significant as it does not always improve reproductive performance.

When should leptospirosis be suspected?

One of the most problematic aspects of leptospirosis is its diagnosis, as the clinical signs are not usually very specific. Leptospirosis should be suspected in the event of:

- Fever, jaundice, and/or nervous signs in piglets <3 months old.
- Piglets that are aborted, mummified, stillborn, or weak and non-viable.
- Endometritis and poor fertility in the sow with cyclic or acyclic returns (28–35 days).

Most infections are subclinical, and the only clinical signs observed are usually reproductive. This makes laboratory diagnosis necessary, as other diseases, such as PRSS, brucellosis, parvovirus, and SMEDI, can develop with similar clinical signs.

Samples sent to the laboratory

Selection of animals to be tested and suitable samples

- Animals with acute signs: jaundice, haemoglobinuria, etc.
- Animals with reproductive problems that have not been treated with antibiotics.
- Fresh foetuses which have not yet started to decay.

Include foetal stomach contents for polymerase chain reaction (PCR).

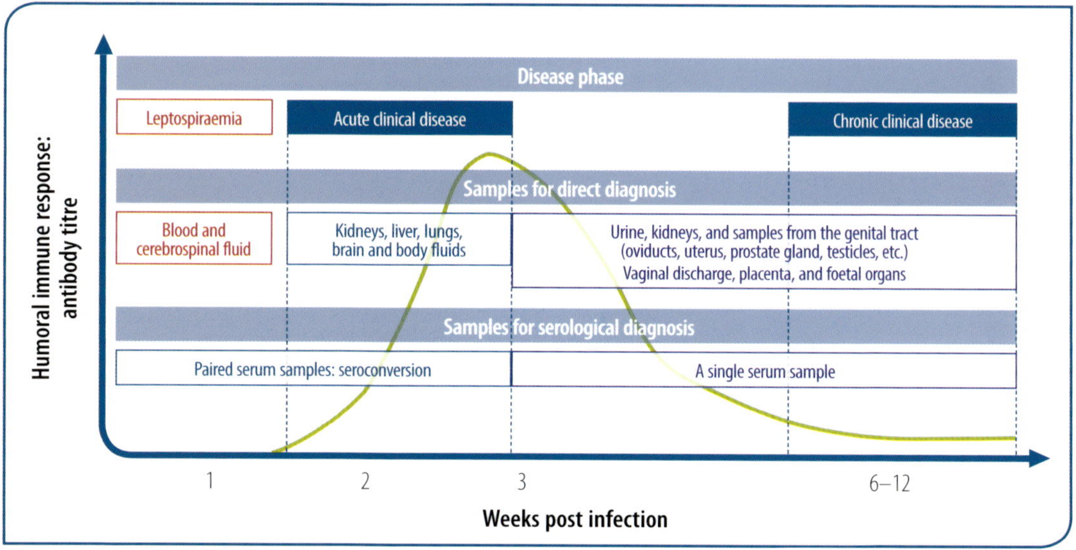

Figure 1. Samples sent to the laboratory according to the clinical signs observed and development of the immune response.

Sending the samples

It is advisable to contact the laboratory where the tests are to be conducted before sending specimens, so that they can advise on the samples to be taken and how to collect, preserve, and transport them, as these requirements depend on the diagnostic tests to be used. The least time possible should elapse between sample collection and arrival at the laboratory.

Table 1. Sample type and transport conditions according to the diagnostic technique used.

Diagnostic technique	Transport medium with serum albumin	Use of swabs	Storage temperature		Immersion in formalin
			25 °C	-20 °C	
Culture	✔	✘	✔	✘	✘
Histology	✘	✘	✔	✘	✔
Immunofluorescence (IF) or immunoperoxidase (IP)	✘	✘	✔	✔	±
PCR	✘	✔	✔	✔	✔
Serology by microagglutination (MAT)	✘	✘	✔	±	✘
Serology by enzyme-linked immunosorbent assay (ELISA)	✘	✘	✔	✔	✘

Laboratory diagnostic methods

Diagnostic methods are classified into 2 broad groups:

- Direct: based on detecting the bacteria themselves, or bacterial antigens, or their nucleic acid.
- Indirect: based on detecting antibodies to infection.

Table 2. Characteristics of the main methods of laboratory diagnosis for leptospirosis.

Characteristic	Direct methods				Serological tests	
	Direct observation	Culture	IF or IP	PCR	MAT	ELISA
Speed	+++	-	+++	+++	+	+++
Sensitivity	-	+++	+	++	++	+
Specificity	-	+++	++	++	+++	++
Difficulty	++	+++	+	-	++	-
Identification of the serogroup involved	-	+++	-	-	++	+

Table 3. Advantages and disadvantages of diagnostic techniques for leptospirosis.

Test	Advantages	Disadvantages
Direct		
Culture	▶ Definitive diagnosis: the only technique that enables the serovar involved to be identified. ▶ Identifies the serovars circulating in a country or region. ▶ Creates a collection of strains for epidemiological and antibiotic resistance studies.	▶ Very dependent on sample quality. ▶ Tedious: up to 6 months for a negative result. ▶ Difficult: contamination, addition of fresh culture medium, etc.
Immunohistochemical tests (IF and IP)	▶ Speed ▶ Useful to diagnose foetal infection and acute cases. ▶ Do not require viable leptospires.	▶ Lack of commercial reagents. ▶ Not very effective in detecting chronic carriers. ▶ Require leptospires that have retained their antigenic integrity.
PCR	▶ Distinguishes between pathogenic and saprophytic leptospires. ▶ Does not require viable or complete leptospires. ▶ Speed, especially real-time PCR (RT-PCR).	▶ Lack of validation for animal tissues. ▶ Proven specificity compared with MAT, but not with culture. ▶ Inhibitors present in the sample, especially in foetal samples. ▶ Does not distinguish between serogroups.

Test		Advantages	Disadvantages
Indirect or serological			
MAT		• Possible to identify the serogroup involved. • Method of reference for international trade. • Useful for individual diagnosis of acute cases, herd diagnosis, and epidemiological studies.	• Storage and testing of strains of live organisms. • Sensitivity depends on the spectrum of serogroups selected. • Individual diagnosis: useful in chronic infections, but of limited use if the disease is caused by strains from the Australis serogroup (Bratislava serovar).
ELISA	Outer membrane proteins (OMPs)	• Reacts to all pathogenic leptospires: useful to diagnose acute infections.	• Validated against MAT in presence of titres of ≥1/100: poor sensitivity for chronic infections. • Does not distinguish between infected and vaccinated animals.
	Outer membrane lipopolysaccharides (LPS)	• Specific to the serogroup: useful in epidemiological studies and monitoring programmes.	

Cell culture is the only test that allows the serovar involved to be identified, but it is a complicated, slow, and tedious procedure. For this reason, it is advisable to:

- Use it in combination with a quick test, immunofluorescence (IF) or PCR, to reach a positive or negative diagnosis of leptospirosis.
- Send serum samples for a microscopic agglutination test (MAT), to determine the serogroup involved. The serogroup will usually be the one with the highest titres. The spectrum of strains that should be selected for MAT are representatives of strains that are adapted to the pig (Bratislava, Pomona, and Tarassovi), and strains that are not adapted but that circulate in the country or region (e.g. the Castellonis, Icterohaemorrhagiae, Canicola, and Hardjo serovars in Spain).

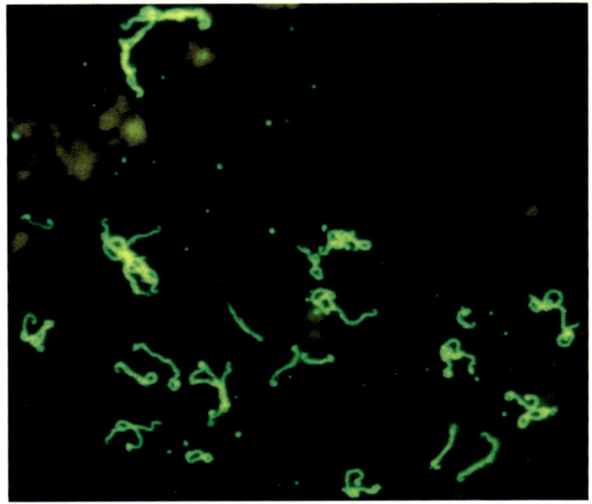

Figure 2. Positive IF for homogenised foetal viscera.

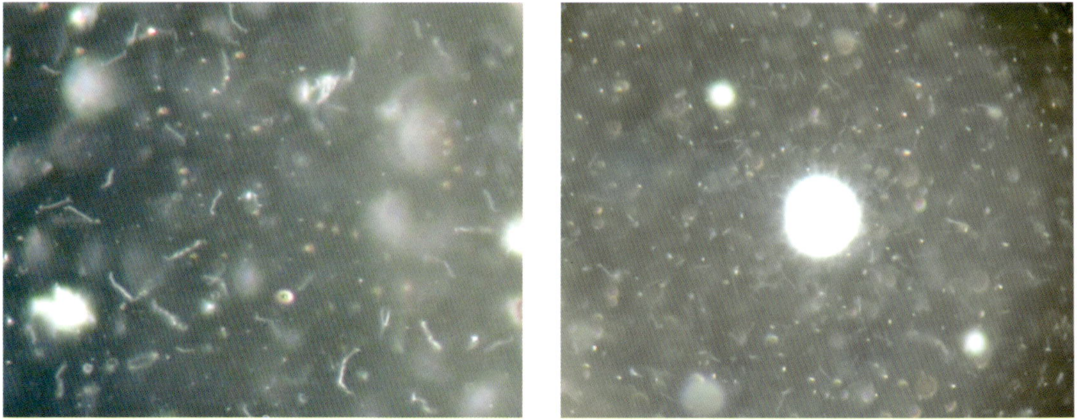

Figure 3. Different degrees of agglutination in a culture of the Pomona serogroup, using MAT.

Objective of diagnosis

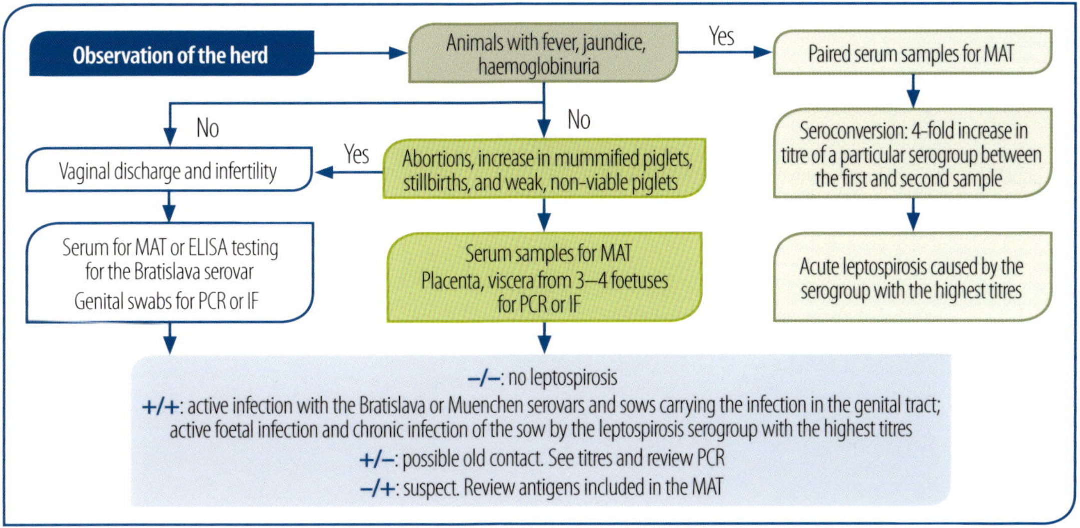

Figure 4. Leptospirosis: diagnosis of the different clinical pictures.

Diagnosis of acute leptospirosis

Acute leptospirosis is caused by infection with some serovars of the Pomona serogroup and accidental serovars (adapted to other species).

Diagnosis is relatively straightforward because a first serum sample can be taken from the affected animals as soon as signs are first seen, and a second at 14–20 days. These paired samples are examined using MAT to detect any seroconversion. The serogroup with the highest titres and most seroconversion is usually the serogroup responsible. If the affected animals have died, there is also usually a large number of leptospires in almost all tissues, and these are easily detected by IF, PCR, and even by cell culture.

However, even if serology is negative for the most common serogroups (Icterohaemorrhagiae, Canicola, Grippotyphosa, Pomona, etc.), leptospirosis disease still cannot be ruled out. Representative strains of all the serogroups would have to be included in the selection of MAT antigens in order to rule out leptospirosis.

Diagnosis of abortions, stillbirths, and non-viable piglets at birth

Samples of the placenta and foetal viscera should be sent to the laboratory. This should be from several foetuses as foetal infection is sequential and not all foetuses may be infected when abortion occurs. Serum from animals that abort, or give birth to small litters or weak, non-viable piglets, should also be submitted.

Diagnosis of accidental serovars is relatively simple: there is a high level of leptospires in foetal tissue, and this is easily detected by IF or PCR. MAT does not detect seroconversion, as the antibody titre has stabilised or may be decreasing when abortion occurs. Despite this, the antibody titre is normally still high (>1/300) when abortion takes place.

Diagnosis is more difficult if reproductive problems are caused by adapted serovars, because there are fewer leptospires in the tissues. However, IF and PCR are still useful for detecting leptospires in foetal tissues. The usefulness of MAT depends on the serogroup/serovar involved:

- Pomona: a high antibody titre is usually detected at the time of abortion.
- Bratislava: MAT is capable of detecting low titres if present. However, no antibodies at all may be found in a third of the animals affected at the time of abortion.

Diagnosis of infertility

Do I have leptospirosis on my farm? If I do, is it active?

Infertility is caused by infection with strains of the Australis serogroup (Bratislava and Muenchen serovars). The main problem in these cases is that immune response to these serovars is poor and titres can drop quickly. It is advisable to consider MAT titres as low as 1/10 to be potential positives in these cases.

Serum from 10 % of the farm's sows, or a minimum of 10 serum samples from farms with <100 animals, should be sent for testing. An equal number of samples should be taken from each group of sows. Serum samples should also be sent from all boars.

The results should be evaluated to determine the serological profile. Infection is considered active if ≥10 % of the animals present with titres ≥1/100. If animals with any detectable antibody titre (≥1/10) are taken to be seropositive, various patterns of infection can be envisaged.

Depending on the results, swabs of any vaginal discharge from repeating sows should be sent to the laboratory, with no transport medium, for PCR.

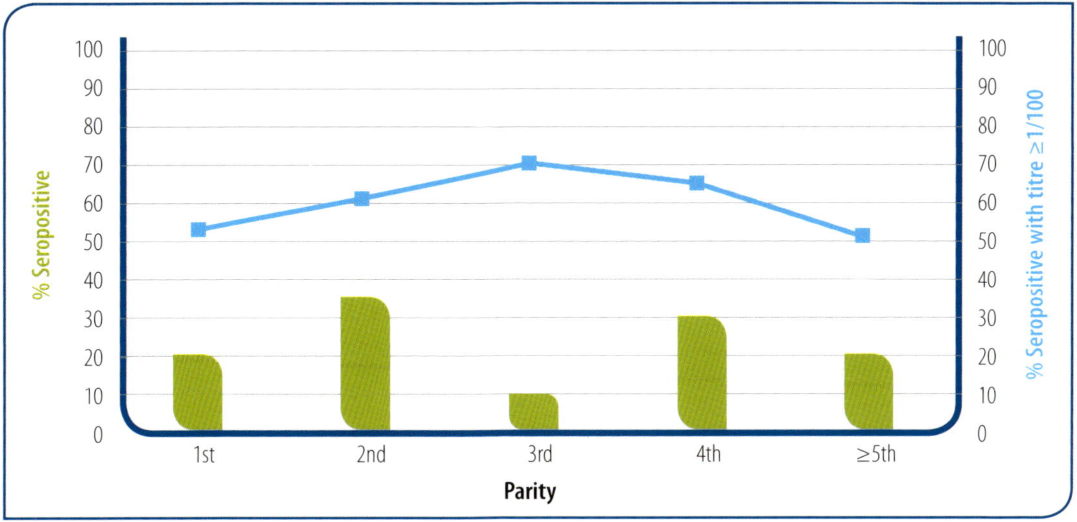

Figure 5. Recent active infection. High percentage of seropositive animals, regardless of parity, a high proportion of which has titres ≥1/100.

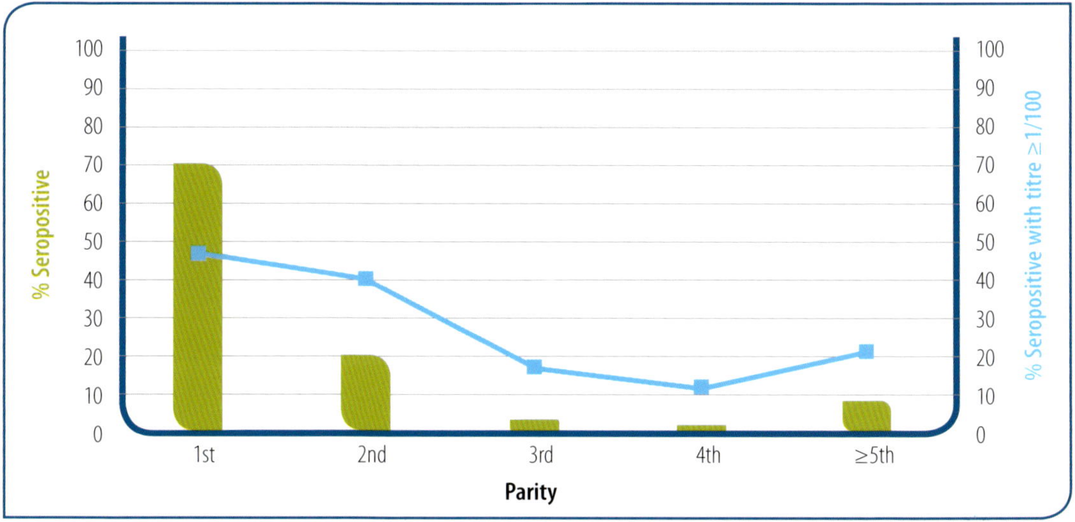

Figure 6. Endemic active infection. High percentage of seropositive animals in first and second parity sows, a high proportion of which has titres ≥1/100.

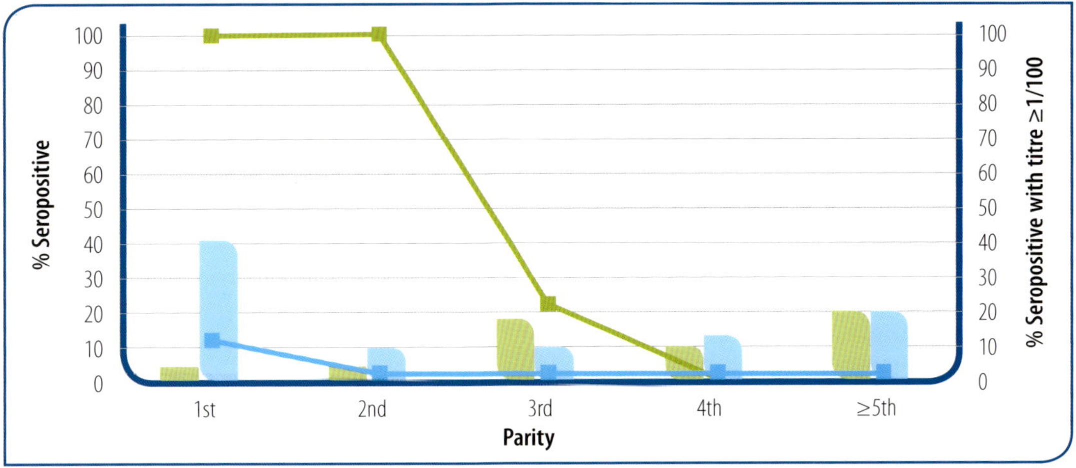

Figure 7. Recent inactive infection. (a) Relatively high percentage of new seropositive sows in the first and second parity groups, while the percentage of animals with titres ≥1/100 is very low. There is a low percentage of seropositive animals in the higher parity groups, and the percentage of animals with titres ≥1/100 is also very low in these groups. (b) Very low percentage of seropositive first and second parity sows, although a high percentage of these has titres ≥1/100. There is a low percentage of seropositive animals in the higher parity groups, and the percentage of animals with titres ≥1/100 is also very low in these groups.

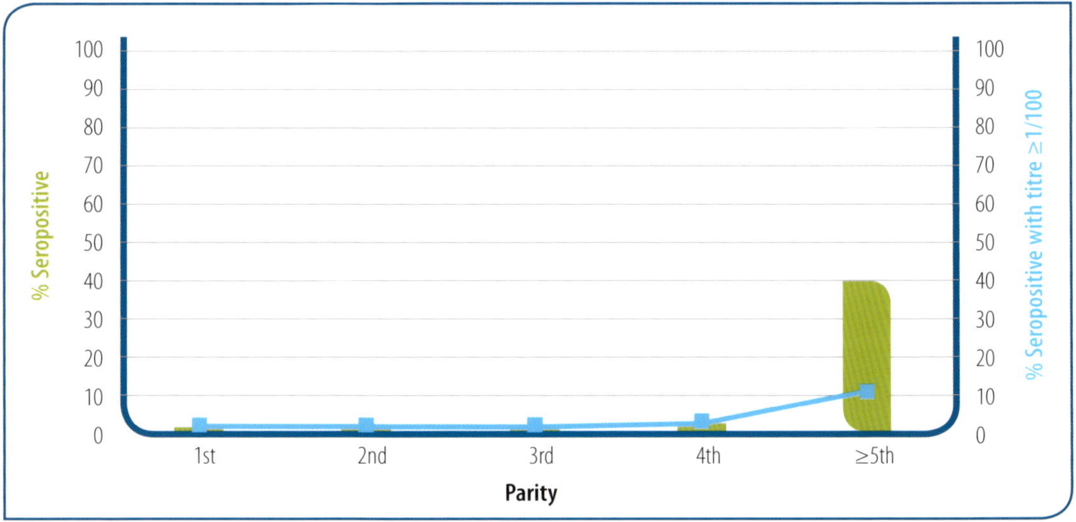

Figure 8. History of chronic infection. Few or no seropositive animals with any number of litters, with a small number of seropositives after the 4th–5th litter.

Interpreting the results

- Acute clinical disease:
  - Detection of leptospires, or their antigens or nucleic acid, in the viscera or body fluids of animals with compatible clinical signs: fever, jaundice, haemoglobinuria, etc.
  - Seroconversion in paired serum samples from animals displaying clinical signs.

- Active foetal infection and probable chronic infection of the dam: detection of leptospires, or their antigens or nucleic acid, in the viscera or body fluids of aborted foetuses, or stillborn or unthrifty piglets.
- Chronic carrier state: detection of leptospires, or their antigens or nucleic acid, in the kidneys, urine or genital tract of animals with no clinical signs, with or without antibodies in their serum.
- Previous contact with the bacteria: detection of antibodies in the serum of animals with reproductive clinical signs, or with no clinical signs, whether carriers or not.

Treatment

Streptomycin, alone or in combination with penicillin, is the treatment of choice. In acute cases with jaundice and haemoglobinuria, affected animals and those at risk of infection should be treated with streptomycin at a dose of 25 mg/kg bodyweight as a single dose or daily over a period of 3–5 days.

In the case of abortions, some studies suggest that antibiotic therapy has little effect on the abortion process once it has started. However, treatment of all sows with 30 mg/kg dihydrostreptomycin has also been reported to stop an abortion outbreak. Additionally, some authors recommend treating all sows with streptomycin or another injectable antibiotic 1 week before insemination and 2 weeks before farrowing to reduce the likelihood of abortions and other reproductive problems.

Other antibiotic treatments that have been used effectively are: ampicillin, amoxicillin, tetracyclines, third-generation cephalosporins, doxycycline, tiamulin and tulathromycin.

Control

Controlling leptospirosis in pigs is based on a combination of 3 strategies: antibiotic therapy, vaccination, and health–hygiene prophylaxis.

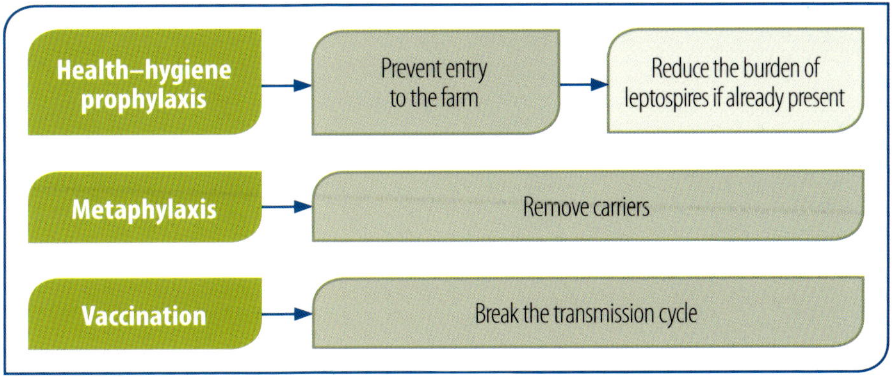

Figure 1. Leptospirosis control strategies and main objectives of each measure.

Health–hygiene prophylaxis

The main measures adopted depend on the farm's current situation.

Farms that are free of infection

The objective in these cases is to prevent infection from entering the farm in contaminated material or infected animals. The key points are:

Semen management

This point is very important for serovar Bratislava, as some strains of this serovar colonise the boar's genital tract and persist there for long periods.

Although no studies have been carried out into how long leptospires can survive in fresh semen or semen treated with non-spermicidal antimicrobial preservatives, survival of 1 month has been reported for bull semen with an appropriate dose of streptomycin and penicillin, so best management practice would be to source semen from pig selection or A.I. centres that are free of the infection.

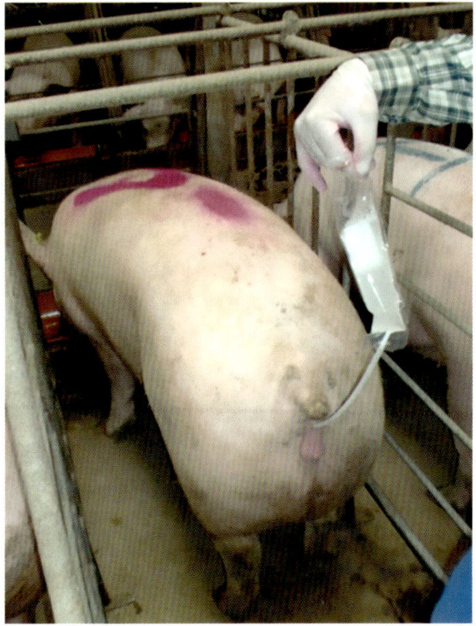

Figure 2. Semen can be an important source of infection during A.I., especially for strains of serovar Bratislava. Image courtesy of Marcial Marcos Cienfuegos.

Quarantine and detection of carrier animals

It is advisable to put animals from other farms, or animals that have been to shows, exhibitions, competitions, etc. through a strict quarantine before they are introduced into the herd. This quarantine should last at least 1 month, but ideally 6 weeks, with appropriate tests being carried out to detect infected animals.

However, this measure is limited by the fact no single test is guaranteed to detect carriers. For example, the reference serological test (MAT) is unreliable as animals infected by host-adapted serovars, especially Bratislava, can be carriers without having any detectable antibodies.

Serological tests can be complemented with PCR tests on urine samples and genital swabs. However, a negative result does not guarantee that the animal is not a carrier, as excretion is intermittent, and for this reason, some authors advise treating quarantined animals with streptomycin.

Prevent contact with other animal species

Different mammalian species can act as maintenance hosts for different serovars. It is particularly important to prevent contact with wild boar, which are a reservoir for strains of serovars Pomona and Bratislava. Hedgehogs, dogs and equines are also maintenance hosts for some serovar Bratislava strains.

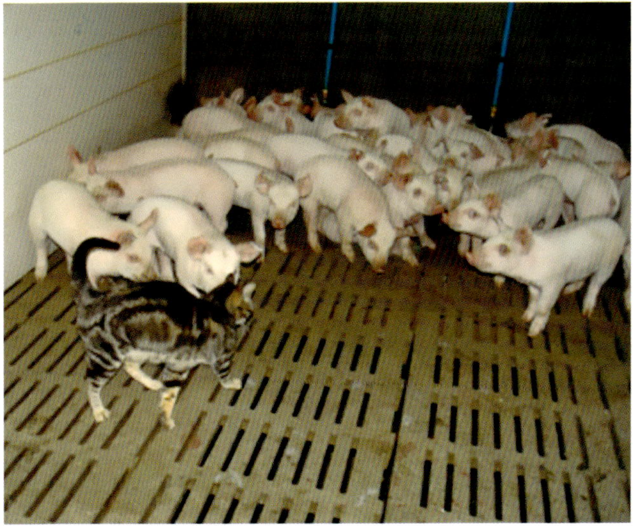

Figure 3. Contact with other domestic animals is a risk factor for infection. Image courtesy of Marcial Marcos Cienfuegos.

From this perspective, it is also extremely important to establish a good rodent control programme, as rodents are a reservoir for a wide range of serovars.

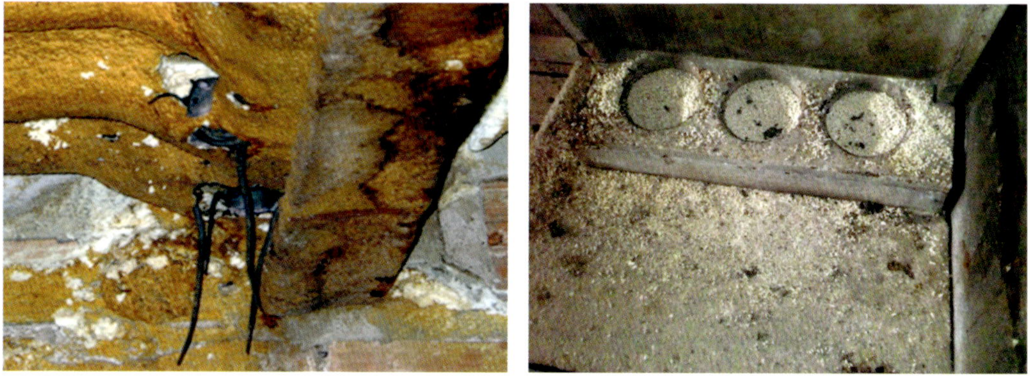

Figure 4. Rodent control is essential, as rodents are a reservoir for many *Leptospira* serovars (e.g., Icterohaemorrhagiae). Images courtesy of Marcial Marcos Cienfuegos.

Ensure that the drinking water supply is clean and free of *Leptospira*

Chlorination, treatment with hydrogen peroxide, or other water purification processes can be used for this. Access by outdoor stock to waterlogged areas where leptospires can survive longer must also be limited.

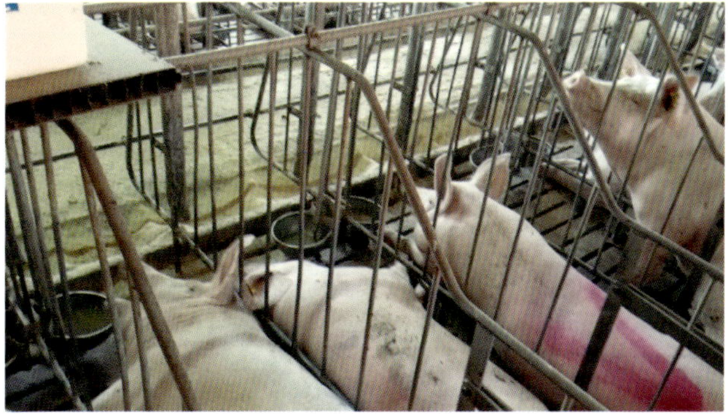

Figure 5. Satisfactory drinking water purification is important to prevent leptospirosis from entering the farm.

Infected farms

The objective in these cases is to ensure that animals are exposed to as low a level of *Leptospira* as possible, so appropriate cleaning, disinfecting and maintenance must be carried out. Floors must be properly concreted and drained for this purpose, to prevent water and urine accumulating.

Cleaning must be regular to prevent accumulation of manure and it is also important to disinfect pens, tools, etc. regularly with suitable products, such as those based on sodium hypochlorite.

Bedding and displaceable materials, such as straw, hay, shavings, etc. should be changed and removed regularly. These materials protect bacteria from environmental conditions and allow leptospires to survive longer in the environment.

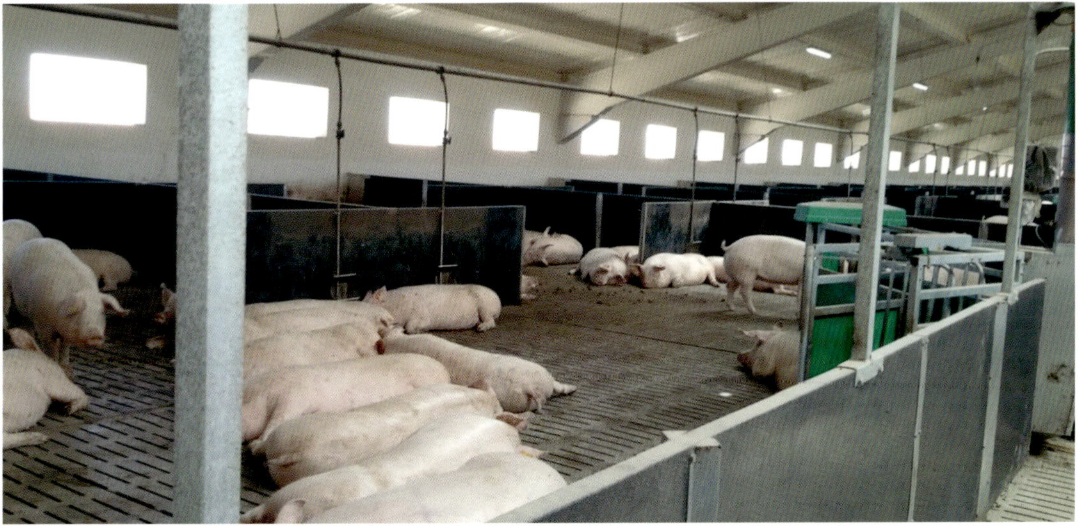

Figure 6. Cleaning, disinfection and adequate drainage are important to reduce the leptospire burden and control their distribution once infection has entered the farm.

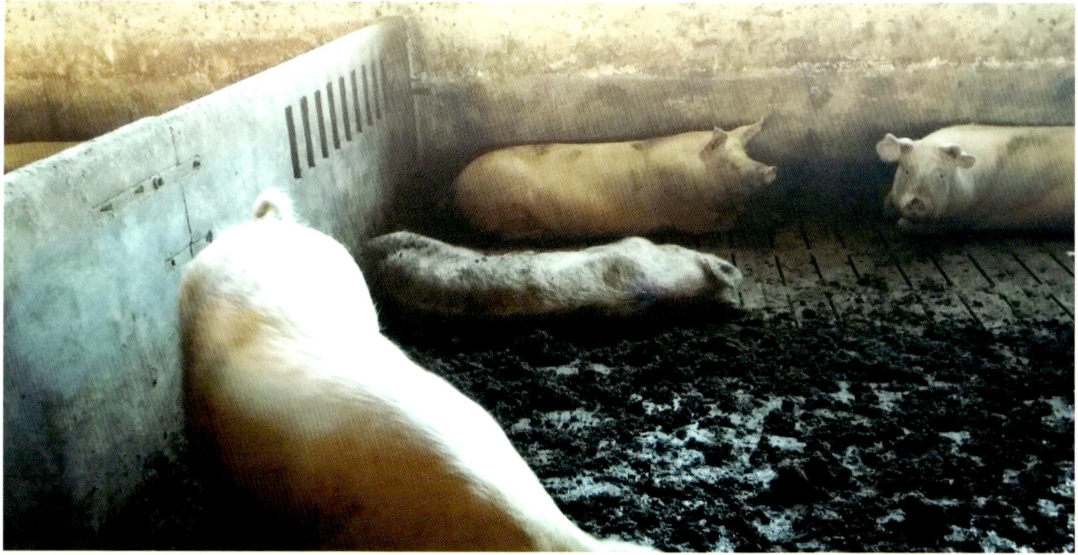

Figure 7. Accumulation of urine and manure encourages leptospire survival on infected farms.

Antibiotic metaphylaxis

Antibiotic therapy has been used as a management tool to reduce the number of carrier animals and minimise levels of circulating leptospires but the serious problems caused by increasing bacterial resistance to antimicrobials and its impact on human health makes this use of antibiotics questionable.

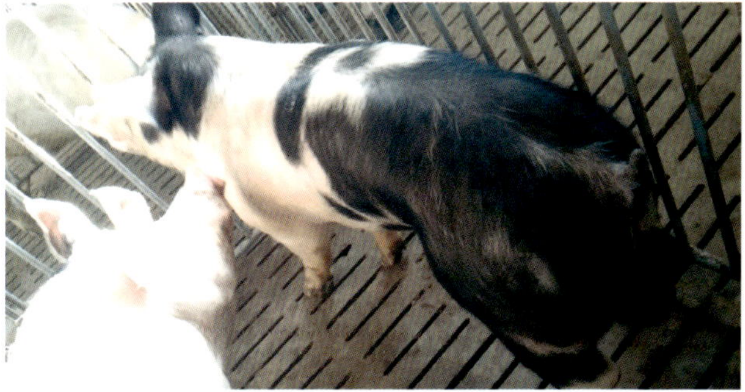

Figure 8. Some authors advise treating boars periodically with streptomycin as part of a control programme.

Control programmes are based on treating all animals on the farm at the same time and then treating any new animals that are subsequently brought onto the farm. A prototype programme would consist of medicating the ration of breeding animals with a suitable level of chlortetracycline or oxytetracycline so that each animal is given a dose of at least 10 mg/kg bodyweight. Rations with 600–800 g antibiotic per tonne of feed are usually used, and these are fed for at least 3 weeks, usually from weaning until 1 month after first insemination. The medicated feed can be combined with individual treatment of all breeding animals with streptomycin at insemination and 14 days after. All boars would also be treated regularly with streptomycin approximately every 6 weeks.

In cases of infertility, some authors have reported an improvement in conception and farrowing rates during the treatment period, but these figures tend to fall again when treatment ends. This, and the issue of antibiotic resistance, suggests that medication should only be used as part of an integrated disease control programme.

Vaccination

The most effective way to control infection is regular and systematic livestock vaccination to break the transmission cycle, although vaccination alone does not eliminate infection. Current commercial products are inactivated bacterial vaccines with different combinations of the serovars that are usually linked to parvovirus and erysipelas.

The vaccines that are generally available include serovars Bratislava, Canicola, Grippotyphosa, Icterohaemorrhagiae and Pomona. These vaccines contain specific serovars, although they do protect relatively well against other serovars in the same serogroup.

In many cases, these vaccines do not protect against renal infection and colonisation, although they reduce but not stop a leptospiruria that has already started. They also do not prevent abortions if the placenta has already been colonised.

Inactivated vaccines

5–7 serovars:

- Specific serovars.
- Relative protection against the serogroup.

Immunity to infection:

- Accidental serovars Pomona and Tarassovi: 1 year.
- Serovar Bratislava: less than 2 pregnancies (6 months).

Immunity to clinical disease:

- Abortion: if the placenta has already been colonised.
- Leptospiruria: continues if it has already started.
- Unknown duration (over 1 year).

Effects on the farm:

- Infection is not eliminated.
- Prevalence is reduced.

Figure 9. Main characteristics of the commercial vaccines used to control leptospirosis in pigs.

Vaccines are considered quite effective in preventing disease caused by accidental serovars and the adapted serovar Pomona, and protection lasts around 12 months, sometimes longer. In the case of serovar Pomona, an abortion rate of 7 % has been reported in sows that have been vaccinated and then challenged after 12 months with strains of the same serovar, compared with 69 % in unvaccinated sows. The incidence of mummified piglets and stillbirths was 13.2 % in the vaccinated sows and 57 % in the control group.

Few efficacy studies have been carried on serovar Bratislava, as isolating strains of this serovar is so difficult. One trial found that pigs vaccinated against serovar Bratislava and challenged experimentally 6 weeks later with a strain of the same serovar developed transient leptospiraemia, but eliminated the infection. However, when challenged 6 months after vaccination, all the animals became infected. The authors concluded that protection is short–lived and covers less than 2 gestations.

With respect to protection against the disease, various trials have reported that vaccination against serovar Bratislava on infected farms significantly improved reproductive parameters.

Farm A		Farm B		Farm C	
Seroprevalence					
64 %		24 %		62 %	
Vaccination					
5 lepto	5 lepto + Bratislava	5 lepto	5 lepto + Bratislava	5 lepto	5 lepto + Bratislava
Effect on some reproductive parameters					
Farrowing rate					
82.7	98.0	78.6	97.2	71.9	94.5
Piglets/litter/sow covered					
6.96	8.82	6.16	8.82	6.95	9.19
Piglets/litter/sow farrowed					
8.42	9.0	7.84	9.07	9.37	9.64

Table 1. Comparison of the effect on some reproductive parameters of vaccination with killed bacterial vaccines that include serovar Bratislava and those that do not (adapted from Frantz et al., 1989).

Autogenous vaccines are an alternative to commercial vaccines, but isolating leptospires is very complicated, especially with strains of the serovar Bratislava. Even if leptospires could be isolated, it would still be difficult to culture enough to produce doses at a sufficiently high concentration of antigen. The use of killed bacterial vaccines produced from reference strains or from strains isolated from other farms, under the name autogenous vaccines, is neither legal nor does it confer anything more than partial protection.

References

Alexopoulos C, Fthenakis GC, Burriel A et al. The effects of the periodical use of in-feed chlortetracycline on the reproductive performance of gilts and sows of a commercial pig with a clinical history of clinical and subclinical viral and bacterial infections. *Reprod Dom Anim*. 2003; 38:87–192.

Arent Z, Frizzell C, Gilmore C et al. *Leptospira interrogans* serovars Bratislava and Muenchen animal infections: implications for epidemiology and control. *Vet Microbiol*. 2016; 190:19–26.

Baker TF, McEwen AS, Prescott JF et al. The prevalence of leptospirosis in association with multifocal interstitial nephritis in swine at slaughter. *Can Vet J*. 1989; 53:290–294.

Bal AE, Gravekamp C, Hartskeerl RA et al. Detection of leptospires in urine by PCR for early diagnosis of leptospirosis. *J Clin Microbiol*. 1994; 32:1894.

Bolin CA, Cassells JA. Isolation of *Leptospira interrogans* serovars bratislava from stillborn and weak pigs in Iowa. *JAVMA*. 1990; 196:1601–1604.

Bolin CA, Cassells JA, Hill HT et al. Reproductive failure associated with Leptospira interrogans serovar bratislava infection of swine. *J Vet Diagn Invest*. 1991; 3:152–154.

Bolin CA, Cassells JA. Isolation of Leptospira interrogans serovars bratislava and hardjo from swine at slaughter. *J Vet Diagn Invest*. 1992; 4:87–89.

Bolin CA. Diagnosis of leptospirosis in swine. *Swine Health Product*. 1994; 2:23–24.

Boqvist S, Chau BL, Gunnarsson A et al. Animal- and herd-level risk factors for leptospiral seropositivity among sows in the Mekong delta, Vietnam. *Prev Vet Med*. 2002; 53:233–245.

Boqvist S, Montgomery JM, Hurst M et al. Leptospira in slaughtered fattening pigs in southern Vietnam: presence of the bacteria in the kidneys and association with morphological findings. *Vet Microbiol*. 2003; 93:361–368.

Chappel RJ, Ellis WA, Adler B et al. Serological evidence for the presence of Leptospira interrogans serovar bratislava in Australian pigs. *Aust Vet J*. 1992; 69:119–120.

Chappel RJ, Prime RW, Millar BD et al. Comparison of diagnostic procedures for porcine leptospirosis. *Vet Microbiol*. 1992; 30:151–163.

Chappel RJ, Prime RW, Millar BD et al. Prevalence and geographic origin of pigs with serological evidence of infection with Leptospira interrogans serovar pomona slaughtered in abattoirs in Victoria, Australia. *Vet Microbiol*. 1998; 62:235–242.

Delbem ACB, de Freitas JC, Bracarense APFRL et al. Leptospirosis in slaughtered sows: serological and histopathological investigation. *Brazilian J Microbiol*. 2002; 33:174–177.

Delbem ACB, Freire RL, da Silva CA et al. Fatores de risco associados à soropositividade para leptospirose em matrizes suínas. *Cienc Rural*. 2004; 34:47–852.

Dikken H, Kmety E. Serological typing methods of leptospires. *Method Microbiol*. 1978; 11:259.

Ellis WA, McParland PJ, Bryson DG et al. Leptospires in pig urogenital tracts and fetuses. *Vet Rec*. 1985; 117:66–67.

Ellis WA, McParland PJ, Bryson DG et al. Prevalence of Leptospira infection in aborted pigs in Northern Ireland. *Vet Rec*. 1986; 118:63–65.

Ellis WA, McParland PJ, Bryson DG et al. Isolation of leptospiras from the genital tract and kidneys of aborted sows. *Vet Rec*. 1986; 118:294–295.

Ellis WA, McParland PJ, Bryson DG et al. Boars as carriers of leptospiras of the Australis serogroup on farms with an abortion problem. *Vet Rec*. 1986; 118:563.

Ellis WA, Thiermann AB. Isolation of Leptospira interrogans serovar bratislava from sows in Iowa. *Am J Vet Res*. 1986; 47:458–460.

Ellis WA, Montgomery JM, McParland PJ. An experimental study with a Leptospira interogans serovar bratislava vaccine. *Vet Rec*. 1989; 125:319–321.

Ellis WA. Leptospirosis. In AD Leman, BE Straw, WL Mengeling, S D´Allaire and DJ Taylor (editors). *Disease of swine*. 7th ed. Iowa University Press. Ames. 1992; pp: 529–536.

Ellis WA, Bolin CA. Leptospirosis. In: *Manual of standards for diagnostic test and vaccines*. Office International de Epizooties (O.I.E.). 1996; p. 198.

Frantz JC, Hanson LE, Brown AL. Effect of vaccination with a bacterin containing Leptospira interrogans serovar bratislava on the breeding performance of swine herds. *Am J Vet Res*. 1989; 50:1044–1047.

García Peña FJ, Fraile L. Leptospira 1: Introduction and pathogenesis. *Int Pig Topics*. 2016; 31 (1).

García Peña FJ, Fraile L. Leptospira 2: Clinical signs and lesions. *Int Pig Topics*. 2016; 31 (2).

García Peña FJ, Fraile L. Leptospira 3: Clinical and laboratory diagnosis–I. *Int Pig Topics*. 2016; 31 (3).

García Peña FJ, Fraile L. Leptospira 4: Clinical and laboratory diagnosis–II. *Int Pig Topics*. 2016; 31 (4).

Gravekamp C, Van de Kemp H, Franzen M et al. Detection of seven species of pathogenic leptospires by PCR using two sets of primers. *J Gen Microbiol*. 1993; 139:1691.

Hathaway SC, Little TWA, Stevens AE. Serological and bacteriological survey of leptospiral infection in pigs in southern England. *Res Vet Sci*. 1981; 31:169-173.

Hathaway SC, Little TWA, Stevens AE. Prevalence and clinical significance of leptospiral antibodies in pigs in England. *Vet Rec*. 1981; 108:224–228.

Hathaway SC, Little TWA, Stevens AE. Isolation of Leptospira interrogans serovar muenchen from a sow with a history of abortion. *Vet Rec*. 1982; 111:100–102.

Hayden H. Leptospira 8: Overall view of leptospira from the UK. *Int Pig Topics*. 2016; 31 (8).

Hayden J. Leptospirosis control in UK pigs. *Vet Rec*. 2000; 147:584.

Hodges RT, Stocker RP, Buddle JR. Leptospira interrogans serotype Pomona infection and leptospiruria in vaccinated pigs. *N Z Vet J*. 1976; 24:37–39.

Hodges RT. *Leptospira interrogans* serotype Pomona infection in pigs: prevention of Leptospiruria by immunisation before exposure to a natural infection. *N Z Vet J*. 1977; 25:33–35.

Jones RT, Millar BD, Chappel RJ et al. Macroscopic kidney lesions in slaughtered pigs are inadequate indicator of current leptospiral infection. *Aust Vet J*. 1987; 64:258–259.

Jung BY, Park CK, Lee CH et al. Seasonal and age-related seroprevalence of Leptospira species in pigs in Korea. *Vet Rec*. 2009; 165:345–346.

Kavanagh N. La experiencia irlandesa y la investigación indican que la descarga vulvar y la L. bratislava se relacionan. *International Pigletter*. 1991; 11:13–14.

Kingscote BF. Leptospirosis outbreak in a piggery in southern Alberta. *Can Vet J*. 1986; 27:188–190.

Lee HS, Khong NV, Xuan HN et al. Sero-prevalence of specific Leptospira serovars in fattening pigs from 5 provinces in Vietnam. *BMC Vet Res*. 2017; 13:125.

Lisboa N. Leptospira 6: Treatment and control. *Int Pig Topics*. 2016; 31 (6).

Little TWA, Hathaway SC. Leptospirosis in pigs. *Vet Ann*, Bristol, England: J Wright & Sons. 1983; 23:116–121.

Michna W. Leptospirosis. *Vet Rec*. 1970; 86:484.

Millán J, Candela MG, López-Bao JV et al. Leptospirosis in wild and domestic carnivores in natural areas in Andalusia, Spain. *Vector-Borne and Zoonotic Dis*. 2009; 9:549.

Miller DA, Wilson MA, Owen WJ et al. Porcine leptospirosis in Iowa. *J Vet Diagn Invest*. 1990; 2:171–175.

Moles-Cervantes LP, Urrutia-Velázquez RM, Diosdado-Vargas F et al. Frecuencia de Leptospira interrogans en unidades de producción porcina del altiplano de México. *Vet Méx*. 1998; 29:49–52.

Mousing J, Christensen J, Haugegaard J et al. A seroepidemiological survey of Leptospira bratislava infections in Danish sow herds. *Prev Vet Med*. 1995; 23:201–213.

Palmer MF. Laboratory diagnosis of leptospirosis. *Med Lab Sci*. 1988; 45:174.

Parma AE, Seijo A, Lucchesi PM et al. Differentiation of pathogenic and non-pathogenic leptospires by means of the polymerase chain reaction. *Rev Inst Med Trop Sao Paulo*. 1997; 39:203.

Perea A, García Gimeno RM, Carranza A et al. Encuesta serológica de leptospirosis en cerdos en la provincia de Badajoz. *Anaporc*. 1991; 98:18–19.